Mediterranean Sweet & Savory Wonders

A Set of Delicious Mediterranean Soups, Breakfast & Dessert Recipes

Valerie Reynolds

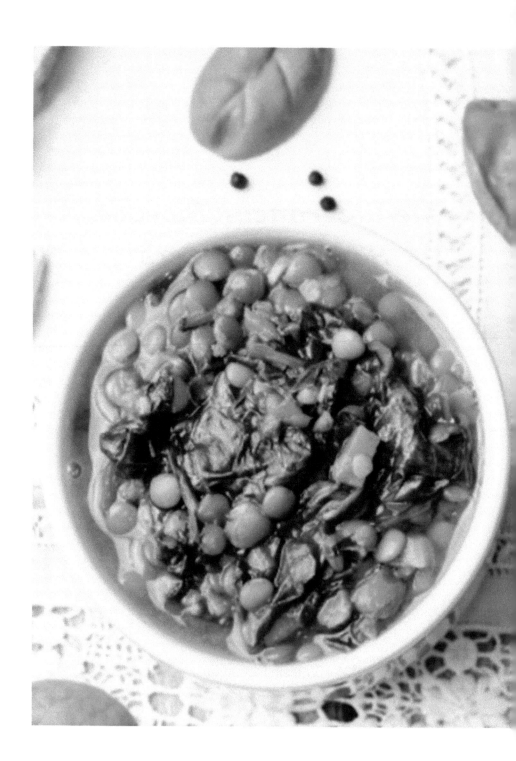

By reading this document, the reader agrees that under no circumstances is the author responsible for any losses, direct or indirect, which are incurred as a result of the use of information contained within this document, including, but not limited to, — errors, omissions, or inaccuracies.

Table of Contents

Mediterranean spicy spinach lentil soup

Ingredients

- 1 large yellow onion, finely chopped
- 1 ½ teaspoons of ground cumin
- 2 teaspoons of dried mint flakes
- Pinch of sugar
- 1 tablespoon of flour
- 6 cups of low-sodium vegetable broth
- 2 cups of chopped flat leaf parsley
- 1 ½ teaspoons of sumac
- Private reserve Greek extra virgin olive oil
- 1 large garlic clove, chopped
- 1 ½ teaspoons of crushed red peppers
- 3 cups of water, more if needed
- 12 ounces of frozen cut leaf spinach
- 1 ½ teaspoons of ground coriander
- Salt and pepper
- 1 ½ cups of green lentils or small brown lentils, rinsed
- 1 lime, juice of lemon

Directions

- In a large ceramic pot, heat 2 tablespoons of olive oil.
- Add the chopped onions and Sauté until golden brown.
- Add the garlic, all the spices, dried mint, sugar, and flour.
- Let cook for 2 minutes on medium heat stirring regularly.
- Add the broth and water.
- Increase the heat to high and boil to a rolling point.
- Add the frozen spinach and the lentils.
- Continue to cook for 5 minutes on high heat.
- Lower the heat and let simmer when covered for 20 minutes.
- Once the lentils are fully cooked, stir in the lime juice and chopped parsley.
- Remove from the heat source and let settle covered for 5 minutes.
- Serve and enjoy hot with pita bread.

Baked eggs with avocado and feta

Ingredients

- salt and fresh-ground black
- Olive oil
- 4 eggs
- 1 avocado
- 2 tablespoons of crumbled feta cheese

Directions

- Break eggs into individual ramekins.
- Let eggs and avocado come to room temperature for 15 minutes.
- Set the oven to 400F.
- Put the gratin dishes on a baking sheet and heat them in the oven for 10 minutes.
- Peel the avocado and cut each half into 6 slices.
- Remove gratin dishes from the oven and spray with olive oil.
- Arrange the sliced avocados in each dish and tip two eggs into each dish.
- Sprinkle with crumbled feta.

- Season to taste with salt and fresh-ground black pepper.
- Let bake for 12 until the whites are set.
- Serve and enjoy hot.

Avocado Caprese wrap

Ingredients

- balsamic vinegar
- 2 whole wheat tortillas
- 1 ball fresh mozzarella cheese sliced
- kosher salt and freshly ground black pepper
- olive oil
- ½ cup of fresh arugula leaves
- 1 tomato sliced
- 1 avocado pitted and sliced
- basil leaves

Directions

- Layer slices of tomato together with the mozzarella cheese and avocado on the tortilla.
- Add a few torn pieces of basil leaves.
- Drizzle with olive oil and balsamic vinegar.
- Season with kosher salt and pepper,
- Fold the tortilla in thirds.
- Serve and enjoy.

Caprese avocado toast

Directions

- Flaked sea salt
- 1 slice whole-wheat toast
- Basil leaves
- 2 teaspoons of flaxseed oil
- 1 small tomato
- ½ avocado, peeled and sliced
- 1/3 cup of low-fat cottage cheese

Directions

- Begin by toasting your bread
- Drizzle with flaxseed oil.
- Layer with the avocado, cottage cheese and tomato.
- Garnish with basil leaves and flaked sea salt.
- Serve and enjoy.

Saucy Greek baked shrimp

Ingredients

- ½ teaspoon of ground cinnamon
- ½ teaspoon of ground allspice
- 1 pound large peeled and deveined shrimp
- ½ teaspoon of red pepper flakes
- ¼ teaspoon of kosher salt
- 2 tablespoons of chopped fresh dill
- 3 tablespoons of olive oil
- ½ cup of crumbled feta cheese
- 3 garlic cloves pressed or minced
- 1 15- ounce can of crushed tomatoes
- 1 medium onion chopped

Directions

- Preheat your oven ready to 375°F.
- Pat dry the shrimp and place in a bowl.
- Season with the red pepper flakes and kosher salt, keep aside.
- Drizzle the olive oil in a heavy skillet and heat over medium heat.

- Add the onion and garlic and cook until softened in 5 minutes.
- Stir in the spices let cook for 30 seconds.
- Add the tomatoes and simmer, uncovered, for about 20 minutes, stirring occasionally.
- Remove from the heat.
- Put shrimp into the tomato sauce and crumble the feta cheese over the top.
- Let bake for 18 minutes until cooked through.
- Sprinkle with the dill.
- Serve and enjoy with crusty bread.

Greek red lentil soup

Trust me, this is a huge surprise to your taste buds. Flavored with onions and garlic and sweetness of the sweet carrots with tomatoes infused with cumin, oregano and rosemary makes this a perfect Mediterranean Sea diet.

Ingredients

- 1 large onion, chopped
- 3 teaspoons of dry oregano
- 1 ½ teaspoons of cumin
- 1 teaspoon of rosemary
- Juice of 2 lemons
- Fresh parsley for garnish
- ½ teaspoon of red pepper flakes
- Extra virgin olive oil
- 2 dry bay leaves
- Crumbled feta cheese to serve
- 7 cups of low-sodium vegetable broth
- 3 garlic cloves, minced
- 2 carrots, chopped
- 2 cups of red lentils , rinsed and drained

- Kosher salt
- 1 cup of crushed tomatoes
- Zest of 1 lemon

Directions

- Heat 3 tablespoons of extra virgin olive oil until shimmering without smoke.
- Add onions, carrots and garlic let cook for 4 minutes, stirring regularly.
- Add spices and bay leaves.
- Cook for a few seconds till fragrant, keep stirring.
- Add crushed tomatoes together with the broth, and lentils.
- Season with kosher salt and boil.
- Reduce the heat let simmer for 20 minutes.
- Remove from heat, let cool then immerse blender to puree.
- Return soup to heat, and stir to warm through.
- Add lemon zest, lemon juice, and fresh parsley.
- Move soup to serving bowls and top with extra virgin olive oil.

- Serve and enjoy.

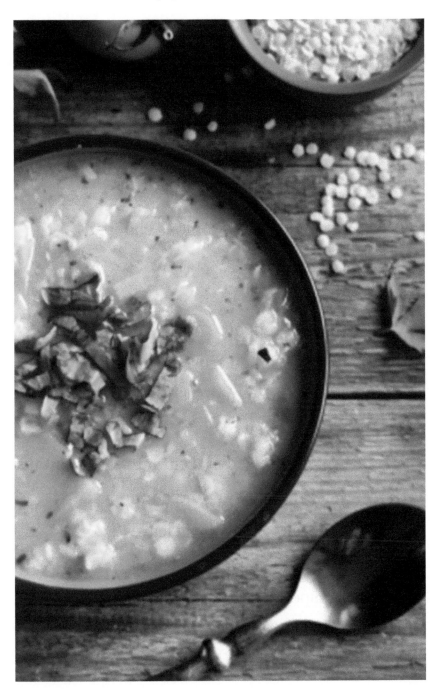

Roasted tomato basil soup

This Mediterranean Sea diet recipe combines aromatic fresh herbs and warm spices. The extra virgin olive oil will give your taste buds the final blast.

Ingredients

- Extra virgin olive oil
- 2 teaspoons of thyme leaves
- 2 medium yellow onions chopped
- Splash of lime juice
- 5 garlic cloves minced
- Salt and pepper
- 1 cup of canned crushed tomatoes
- 3 lb.. Roma tomatoes halved
- 2 ½ cups of water
- 3 carrots peeled and cut into small chunks
- ½ teaspoon of ground cumin
- 2 ounces of fresh basil leaves
- 4 fresh thyme springs
- 1 teaspoon of dry oregano
- ½ teaspoon of paprika

Directions

- Heat your oven to 450°F.
- In a large mixing bowl, combine tomatoes and carrot pieces.
- Add a drizzle of extra virgin olive oil, and season with kosher salt and black pepper. Toss.
- Transfer to a large baking sheet and spread well in one layer.
- Roast in heated oven for about 30 minutes.
- Let cool for 10 minutes when ready.
- Transfer the roasted tomatoes and carrots to the large bowl of a food processor fitted with a blade.
- Add just a tiny bit of water and blend.
- In a large cooking pot, heat 2 tablespoons of extra virgin olive oil over medium heat until shimmering without smoke.
- Add onions let cook for 3 minutes.
- Add garlic and cook briefly until golden.
- Pour the roasted tomato mixture into the cooking pot.

- Stir in crushed tomatoes with water, basil, thyme, and spices.
- Season with a little kosher salt and black pepper.
- Boil, then reduce the heat and cover part-way.
- Let simmer for 20 minutes.
- Remove the thyme springs and transfer tomato basil soup to serving bowls.
- Serve and enjoy with lime juice if you desire.

Creamy roasted carrot soup with ginger

The combination of ginger and garlic in one recipe just pulls off the flavor side of it making it a perfect Mediterranean diet recipe. It is gluten free.

Ingredients

- 1 teaspoon of ground coriander
- 3 lb. carrots peeled
- 1 teaspoon of allspice
- Fresh mint
- 1 ½ cup unsweetened half and half
- Greek extra virgin olive oil
- Salt and pepper
- 1 teaspoon of grated fresh ginger
- 5 ½ cups low-sodium vegetable broth divided
- 4 garlic cloves chopped

Directions

- Preheat your oven ready to 425°F.
- Organize the carrots on a large lightly oiled sheet pan.
- Season lightly with salt and pepper and drizzle generously with olive oil.

- Roast in the oven for 45 minutes, turn over mid-way through.
- When the carrots are ready, set aside briefly.
- Cut the carrots into chunks and place them in a large food processor with the garlic, ginger and broth.
- Puree until the mixture is smooth.
- Transfer the carrot puree to a heavy cooking pot.
- Add the remaining broth, coriander and allspice.
- Place the pot on medium heat let boil as you watch. Stir occasionally.
- Reduce the heat to low, stir in the heavy cream to heat through.
- Transfer to serving bowls and garnish with fresh mint leaves.
- Serve and enjoy with rustic bread.

Mediterranean bean soup recipe with tomato pesto

Ingredients

- 1 Large russet potato, peeled, diced
- 2 cups of cooked chickpeas
- 1 15-oz. can of diced tomatoes
- ½ cup grated Parmesan cheese
- 1 tablespoon of ground coriander
- 1 teaspoon of Spanish paprika
- 5 cups of low sodium vegetable broth
- 8-oz. of frozen spinach, no need to thaw
- 2 cups of cooked red kidney beans
- 1 tablespoon of white vinegar
- Basil leaves
- ⅓ cup of toasted pine nuts for garnish
- 1 medium yellow onion, chopped
- Salt and pepper
- 3 large garlic cloves
- Greek extra virgin olive oil
- 2 cups of cooked cannellini beans
- 1 ½ cup of diced fresh tomatoes

- 15 large basil leaves

Directions

- In a large oven, heat 2 tablespoons of olive oil.
- Add the diced potatoes and onions over low heat and let cook for 5 minutes, toss.
- Add tomatoes, vinegar, spices, salt and pepper. Stir.
- Continue to cook for 4 minutes.
- Add vegetable broth with frozen spinach.
- Increase the heat to medium boil for 4 minutes.
- Add the kidney beans together with the cannellini beans, and chickpeas.
- Boil again, then reduce heat to low let cook for 20 minutes.
- In the bowl of a food processor, place garlic and tomatoes.
- Blend briefly to combine.
- Add basil and puree.
- Drizzle in the olive oil a little bit at a time as the processor is still running.

- Transfer the thick tomato pesto to a bowl, and stir in grated Parmesan.
- Stir in the tomato pesto when soup is ready.
- Transfer to serving bowl then top each bowl with a few basil leaves and toasted pine nuts.
- Serve and enjoy with crusty bread.

Mushroom barley soup

Ingredients

- 1 cup of pearl barley rinsed
- Kosher salt
- 1 yellow onion, chopped
- 6 cups of low-sodium broth
- ½ cup of packed chopped parsley
- 2 celery stalks, chopped
- 1 carrot, chopped
- 8 oz.. of white mushrooms, cleaned and chopped
- ½ cup of canned crushed tomatoes
- Black pepper
- 1 teaspoon of coriander
- 4 garlic cloves, chopped
- Extra virgin olive oil
- ½ teaspoon of to 3/4 teaspoon of smoked paprika
- 16 oz. of baby Bella mushrooms
- ½ teaspoon of cumin

Directions

- In a large Oven, heat extra virgin olive oil over medium heat until shimmering without smoke.
- Add baby bell mushrooms let cook until mushrooms are soft.
- Remove from the pot, keep for later.
- In the same pot, add a little more extra virgin olive oil.
- Add onions together with the garlic, carrots, celery, and chopped white mushrooms.
- Cook for 5 minutes over medium-high heat.
- Then, season with salt and pepper.
- Add the crushed tomatoes and spices let cook for 3 minutes, toss regularly.
- Add broth and pearl barley give it a rolling boil for 5 minutes.
- Lower the heat and let simmer over low heat for 45 minutes until the barley is tender.
- Add the cooked Bella mushrooms back to the pot and stir to combine.
- Continue to cook for 5 minutes.

- Add fresh parsley.
- Serve and enjoy.

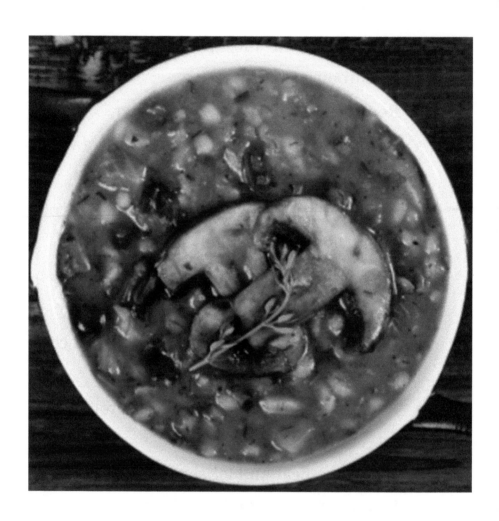

Pressure pot chickpea soup

The chickpea soup is another loaded recipe with variety of vegetables and fresh herbs as well as warm spices. It is gluten free, low carb yet high plant protein based.

Ingredients

- 1 yellow onion, chopped
- 15 oz. can of chopped tomatoes with juice
- 3 garlic cloves, minced
- Salt
- 6 cups low-sodium vegetable broth
- 2 carrots, chopped
- 1 green bell pepper, cored, chopped
- 1 oz. chopped fresh cilantro
- 4 red chili peppers
- 1 teaspoon of ground coriander
- 1 teaspoon of ground cumin
- 2 cups dry chickpeas
- 1 teaspoon of Aleppo pepper
- 1 lemon, juice of
- ½ teaspoon of ground turmeric
- ½ teaspoon of ground allspice

- Greek extra virgin olive oil

Directions

- Place chickpeas in a large bowl and add plenty of water and let soak overnight.
- Preheat your pressure Pot by selecting the Sauté function and adjust heat to high.
- Add 2 tablespoon of extra virgin olive oil let heat until shimmering.
- Add onions together with the garlic and a pinch of salt let cook for 3 minutes, stirring regularly.
- Add carrots, bell peppers, and spices. Continue to cook for 4 minutes, stir to soften the vegetables.
- Add drained chickpeas together with the tomatoes, and broth.
- Lock your pressure Pot lid in place.
- Select the pressure cooking setting and set on high.
- Set the timer to 15 minutes.
- Allow time to let pressure release naturally when cooked.

- Unlock and remove the lid.
- Stir in lemon juice and fresh cilantro.
- Taste and adjust accordingly.
- Transfer to serving bowls and drizzle extra virgin olive oil.
- Serve and enjoy with crusty bread.

Mediterranean bean soup with tomato pesto

Beans are a reliable source of proteins, therefore combined with a variety of vegetables especially tomatoes, it can feed a crowd.

Ingredients

- 1 15-oz. can of diced tomatoes
- 1 tablespoon of white vinegar
- 3 large garlic cloves
- 1 tablespoon of ground coriander
- 1 Large russet potato, peeled, diced into small cubes
- 1 teaspoon of Spanish paprika
- ½ cup of grated Parmesan cheese
- Salt and pepper
- 5 cups of low sodium vegetable broth
- Greek extra virgin olive oil
- 8-oz. of frozen spinach, no need to thaw
- 20 large basil leaves
- 2 cups of cooked red kidney beans
- 1 ½ cup diced fresh tomatoes

- 1 medium yellow onion, chopped
- 2 cups of cooked cannellini beans
- 2 cups of cooked chickpeas
- Basil leaves for garnish
- ⅓ cup of toasted pine nuts for garnish

Directions

- In a heavy pot, heat 2 teaspoons of olive oil.
- Reduce heat to medium and add the diced potatoes and onions let cook for 5 minutes, tossing regularly.
- Add tomatoes together with the vinegar, spices, salt and pepper. Stir to combine.
- Let cover for 4 minutes.
- Add vegetable broth and frozen spinach.
- Increase the heat to medium let boil for 4 minutes.
- Add the kidney beans, cannellini beans, and chickpeas.
- Bring back to a boil.
- Lower the heat cover let cook for 20 minutes.
- In the bowl of a food processor, place garlic and tomatoes.

- Pulse briefly to combine.
- Then, add basil and puree and drizzle in the olive oil a little bit as the processor is still running.
- Transfer the thick tomato pesto to a bowl, stir in grated Parmesan.
- Remove from heat source. Stir in the tomato pesto.
- Shift to the serving bowl.
- Top each bowl with a few basil leaves and toasted pine nuts.
- Serve and enjoy.

Cream of a roasted cauliflower soup with Mediterranean twist

Ingredients

- 2 teaspoons of ground cumin
- Greek extra virgin olive oil
- 1/4 teaspoon of ground turmeric
- Salt and pepper
- ½ lemon, juice of lemon
- 2 ½ cups of fat-free half and half
- 1 small sweet onion, chopped
- 5 garlic cloves, chopped
- 2 heads of cauliflower, cut into florets
- 1 cup chopped fresh dill
- 2 ½ teaspoon of Sweet Spanish paprika
- 4 cups of low-sodium vegetable broth
- 1 cup of water
- 1 teaspoon of ground sumac

Directions

- Start by preheating your oven to 425°F.
- Place cauliflower florets on a large sheet pan.

- Sprinkle with salt and pepper and drizzle with extra virgin olive oil. Toss.
- Spread evenly on sheet pan let roast 45 minutes in the oven, make sure to turn midway to balance the sides.
- In a large heavy pot, heat 2 tablespoons of olive oil until shimmering but without smoke.
- Add onions and let sauté, over medium heat, until translucent.
- Add chopped garlic and spices.
- Stir briefly until fragrant.
- Add 3/4 the amount of roasted cauliflower.
- Stir to coat well with the spices, then add vegetable broth and water.
- Boil, then lower heat to medium.
- Cover part-way and let simmer for 7 minutes.
- Remove from heat.
- Blend cauliflower and liquid until you achieve desired smoothness.
- Return to a medium heat and stir in the fat-free half and half, and lime juice.

- Stir in the remainder of roasted cauliflower florets you reserved earlier.
- Let cook briefly to warm through.
- Test and adjust salt accordingly.
- Stir in the chopped dill.
- Serve and enjoy hot with crusty whole wheat bread.

Curried red lentil and sweet potato soup

Ingredients

- 1 large sweet potato, peeled, cubed
- 1 teaspoon of paprika
- 3 15-oz. cans of vegetable broth
- 1 ½ cup of red lentils, rinsed
- 2 celery ribs, chopped
- 1 large red onion, halved, divided
- 1 teaspoon of mild yellow curry
- Olive oil
- 1 teaspoon of seasoned salt
- 1 bay leaf
- 4 garlic cloves, chopped
- 1 1/4 cup of heavy cream

Directions

- In a non-stick pan, heat a tablespoon of olive oil.
- Sauté sliced onions on medium-high until fairly brown and crispy.
- Remove onions onto a paper towel to drain any excess oil.

- In a large pot, heat 3 tablespoons of olive oil.
- Add chopped onions together with the sweet potato and celery let sauté on medium-high for 5 minutes as you stir infrequently.
- Add garlic, curry, seasoned salt, paprika and bay leaf. Toss toss.
- Pour in three cans of vegetable broth let cook on medium-high and bring to a boil.
- As broth is boiling, stir in rinsed red lentils.
- Let continue to cook for 4 minutes on medium-high heat, stirring occasionally.
- Lower the heat to medium-low, cover let cook for 7 minutes, stirring occasionally.
- Test and adjust accordingly.
- Stir in heavy cream and let cook briefly to warm through.
- Serve and enjoy with browned and crispy onions.

Easy vegan pumpkin soup

Ingredients

- 2 medium yellow onions, chopped
- ½ teaspoon of organic ground turmeric
- Jalapeno slices for garnish
- 2 garlic cloves, minced
- 1/4 cup pine nuts, toasted in olive oil
- 1 teaspoon of organic ground coriander
- 1 cup of red lentils
- 15 oz. can pumpkin puree
- 3 ½ cups quality vegetable broth
- Salt
- 3 tablespoons of gold raisins
- Extra virgin olive oil
- ½ fresh lemon, juice of
- 1 tablespoon of tomato paste
- 1 Zhoug cilantro pesto
- 1 teaspoon of organic ground cumin

Directions

- Prepare your Zhoug spicy cilantro paste normally. Keep aside for later.

- In a heavy pot, heat 2 extra virgin olive oil over medium-high heat until shimmering but without smoke.
- Add the onions let cook until golden and translucent then toss.
- Stir in garlic together with the tomato paste, coriander, cumin, and turmeric.
- Lower heat to medium let cook for 4 minutes, stirring regularly.
- Add the lentils together with the pumpkin puree, broth and a little salt. Stir.
- Raise the heat to high let boil for 5 minutes.
- Then, lower the heat cover only part-way let continue to cook for 20 minutes, stir.
- Remove from heat let cool briefly.
- Transfer the lentil pumpkin soup to the bowl of a large food processor blend.
- Return to pot over medium heat to warm through, stirring occasionally.
- Stir in raisins together with the fresh lemon juice.
- Let cook for 4 minutes, stir regularly.

- Taste adjust accordingly.
- Divide the lentil pumpkin soup into serving bowls.
- Then, top with a teaspoon of Zhoug spicy cilantro pesto and toasted pine nuts.
- Garnish with jalapeno slices, serve.
- Enjoy.

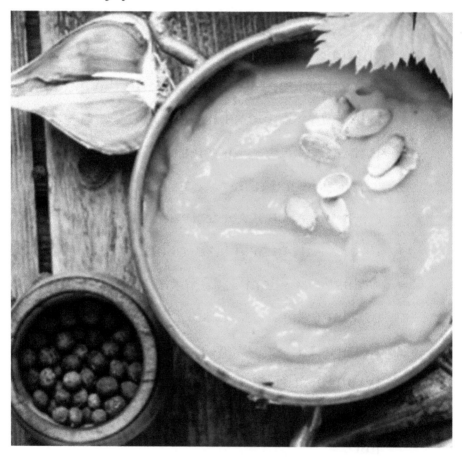

Herbed vegan potato leek soup

Ingredients

- Salt and pepper
- 6 garlic cloves, peeled
- 1 teaspoon of ground cumin
- 1 cup of fresh cilantro leaves
- 1 teaspoon of sweet paprika
- Greek extra virgin olive oil
- Lemon wedges to serve
- 3 leeks, well-cleaned
- 2 dried bay leaves
- 2 lb. Yukon gold potatoes
- 6 cups of vegetable broth

Directions

- In a small food processor, blend garlic cloves and fresh cilantro until finely ground into a paste.
- In a large heavy cooking pot, heat 3 tablespoon of olive oil over medium-high heat until shimmering but with no smoke.

- Add the garlic and cilantro mixture together with the chopped leeks.
- Let cook as you toss regularly, until leeks are tender.
- Add potatoes together with the spices, and a generous dash of salt and pepper. Toss.
- Add the bay leaves and vegetable broth.
- Boil for 5 minutes after which lower the to medium and let simmer for another 15 minutes until the potatoes are tender.
- Turn off heat.
- Fish the bay leaves out.
- Using an immersion blender, blend the potato leek to your liking.
- Place the pot back on stove to heat the soup through over medium heat, stirring.
- Taste and adjust seasoning accordingly.
- Transfer soup to serving bowls.
- Add a generous drizzle of olive oil.
- Serve with lemon wedges and crusty bread.
- Enjoy.

Pressure pot stuffed pepper soup

This a true fuss-free recipe using a pressure pot with two secret ingredients. It derives its taste from variety of flavors.

Ingredients

- 3 cups of beef broth
- 1 onion
- 2 teaspoons of dried oregano
- 1 pound of lean ground beef
- 1 teaspoon of salt
- 3 garlic cloves, minced
- 1 large green bell pepper
- 1½ cup of roasted peppers, drained
- 2 cups of tomato juice
- 1 tablespoon of sunflower oil
- 2 cups of water
- A pinch of black pepper
- ½ cup of uncooked rice

Directions

- Turn on the pressure pot.
- Click Sauté then add oil in.

- Sauté green pepper and onion for 3 minutes
- Add ground beef and minced garlic.
- Break up the meat into smaller pieces.
- Mix.
- Add roasted peppers and the rest of the ingredients.
- Mix well, lock the lid in position.
- Turn the steam valve to sealing.
- Set time to 5 minutes in the manual and let it run.
- When the time is up wait for extra 10 minutes.
- Release the pressure.
- Taste and season accordingly.

Easy geek lentil soup

This recipe leads to a creamy outcome which, by all means will surprise one's taste buds especially when combined with sweet carrots, onions and garlic. More so, it is infused with oregano, rosemary, and oregano to increase your lust for it. It is imperative to not that lentils are one of the vital part of a Mediterranean Sea diet and several other legumes.

Ingredients

- 2 dry bay leaves
- 1 teaspoons of rosemary
- 1 ½ teaspoons of cumin
- 1 large chopped onion
- 2 carrots, chopped
- Extra virgin olive oil
- 3 teaspoons of dry oregano
- Crumbled feta cheese
- 1 cup crushed tomatoes
- Fresh parsley for garnish
- 2 cups red lentils , rinsed and drained
- ½ teaspoons of red pepper flakes

- 3 minced garlic cloves
- Zest of 1 lemon
- Juice of 2 lemons
- Kosher salt
- 7 cups low-sodium vegetable broth

Directions

- Heart about 3 tablespoon of extra virgin oil, endure it does not smoke.
- Add carrots, garlic, and the onions and cook for 3 – 4 minutes while stirring frequently.
- Introduce the bay leaves and spices, then while stirring, cook for a few seconds till fragrant.
- Combine lentils, tomatoes, and the broth and add together, use salt to season.
- Bring it to boil, reduce the heat to allow it to simmer for 15 – 20 minutes.
- Reduce the content from the heat source. Cool off and puree in a blender.
- Pulse until visible cream consistency.
- Place the soup back on heat, continue to stir to allow even warming.
- Introduce the lemon juice and parsley.

- Transfer the soup to serving dishes, of course topped with extra virgin olive oil.
- Serve with crusty bread of your choice and enjoy.

Easy salmon soup

In just 20 minutes or less, this delicacy of creamy chunks of salmon tucked with incredible flavors typical in the broth with carrots and dill. The application of lemon juice brings out the taste in this salmon soup.

Ingredients

- 1 teaspoon of dry oregano
- 1 carrot, thinly sliced into rounds
- Zest and juice of 1 lemon
- 4 green onions, chopped
- 3/4 teaspoon of ground coriander
- 4 garlic cloves, minced
- ½ green bell pepper, chopped
- ½ teaspoon of ground cumin
- Kosher salt and black pepper
- 5 cups low-sodium chicken broth
- 1 ounces of fresh dill, divided, chopped
- Extra virgin olive oil
- 1 lb. gold potatoes, thinly sliced into rounds
- 1 lb. salmon skinless fillet, cut into large chunks

Directions

- In a large pot, heat 2 tablespoons of extra virgin olive oil, allow it to shimmer without smoking.
- Add the bell pepper, garlic, and onions, cook over medium temperature with constant stirring to produce fragrance in 3 minutes.
- Introduce ½ of the fresh dill, then stir for 30 minutes.
- It is time to add the broth, carrots, and potatoes.
- Add the spices, then season with the kosher salt and black pepper.
- Boil in a high temperature, reduce the temperature to medium and continue to cook for 5 – 6 minutes.
- Separately, season the salmon with kosher salt and then introduce it to the pot of soup. Reduce the temperature cook shortly for 3 – 5 minutes to allow the salmon to cook completely.

- Add and stir in the zest, remaining dill, and lemon juice
- Transfer your soup to a serving bowl.
- Serve and enjoy with some crusty breads.

Breakfast egg muffins

These easy to freeze low-carb eggs muffins are a perfect choice of breakfast for anyone who eats eggs. It is even tastier when serves along with veggies and other salads especially the Mediterranean favorite veggies and salads.

Ingredients

- ½ teaspoon of Spanish paprika
- 1 chopped shallot
- 1 28. 34 g chopped fresh parsley leaves
- 1 small chopped red bell pepper
- 8 large eggs
- 12 cherry tomatoes, halved
- 3 to 4 113 g boneless shredded cooked chicken or turkey
- Salt and Pepper
- Extra virgin olive oil for brushing
- Handful crumbled feta to your liking
- 1/4 teaspoon of ground turmeric (optional)
- 6 to 10 pitted Kalamata olives, chopped

Directions

- Get a rack, place it in the middle of your oven and start by preheating it to 350°
- Prepare a muffin pan that can fit 12 muffin cups then brush it all with extra olive oil.
- Equally divide the tomatoes, shallots, chicken, olives, peppers, extra virgin oil, and parsley.
- Add the salt, pepper, eggs, and spices in one bowl, then whisk to allow it combine well.
- Over each of the cups, pour the mixture of eggs, with a small space at the top.
- Place the muffin pan on top of the sheet pan.
- Bake it for approximately 25 minutes in a heated oven.
- Allow it to cool for some time and run some butter along the edges of every muffin.
- Remove it off the pan
- Serve and enjoy

Coconut mango overnight oats

This is high energy giving recipe is ideal for families that are quite busy and always on the go. It is fuss free make with mangoes, oats, coconut and other as listed among the ingredients

Ingredients

- 2 teaspoons of shredded coconut
- A pinch of salt
- 2 teaspoons of honey
- ½ cup of diced mango, frozen or fresh
- ½ cup of milk
- 1 teaspoon of chia seeds
- ½ Cup of rolled oats

Directions

- Start by putting the oats in a jug.
- Add a pinch of salt.
- Pour the over milk over the oats in the jar together with all the other ingredients. Blend well.
- Pack in a closed container and refrigerate overnight.

- Served chilled and enjoy.

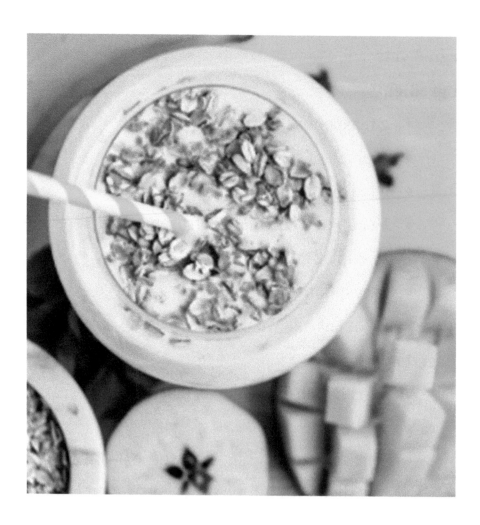

Turmeric hot chocolate

The turmeric hot chocolate has anti-inflammatory properties making a healthier Mediterranean Sea diet choice for anyone.

Ingredients

- 2 teaspoons of honey
- A pinch of cayenne pepper
- 2 teaspoons of coconut oil
- 1 cup of milk
- 1 teaspoon of ground turmeric
- A pinch of black pepper
- 1½ tablespoons of cocoa powder

Directions

- Firstly, place your milk in a sauce pan.
- Then, add turmeric, cocoa powder, and coconut oil.
- Whisk to combine everything.
- Bring to a boil.
- Add black pepper and cayenne pepper when the heat is off, stir.
- Pour in a mug.

- Allow the mixture to cool.
- Then add adding honey.
- Serve and enjoy warm.

Fir tart

Figs fruits are the essential ingredients in making this recipe. It blends puff pastry and ricotta along with fig filling. This recipe is perfect for a Mediterranean desert in about 25 minutes.

Ingredients

- 1 puff of pastry sheet, thawed
- 8 ounces of ricotta
- 3 tablespoons of honey
- 12 fresh figs
- 4 tablespoons of almonds , roughly chopped
- 2 teaspoons of shredded coconut

Directions

- Preheat your oven to 400°F.
- Mix ricotta together with the honey and figs flesh until well combine in a small dish. Keep for later.
- Unfold the pastry and roll it out thin.
- Cut in half.
- Place all of them onto a baking tray aligned with baking parchment.

- Cut indentations alongside the edges.
- Between the two tarts, divide the ricotta mixture and spread over. Make sure the mixture is only in the inner frame cut with the knife.
- Then cut 2 figs into wedges.
- Put them on the tart randomly.
- Then, put the tray in the oven.
- At 400°F, bake for 12 minutes, the edges should become puffed and the bottom should turn golden brown.
- Cut each fig into 8 pieces.
- The almonds should be roughly chopped.
- Take the tarts out when they are ready.
- Use the fresh figs for topping, then sprinkle with almonds and coconut.
- Serve and enjoy warm.

Blueberry turnovers

The recipe combines puff pastry together with homemade blueberry fillings. This Mediterranean diet is fit for breakfast, lunch or dinner.

Ingredients

- All-purpose flour, for dusting
- ⅓ cup brown sugar
- 1 tablespoon lemon juice
- 1 teaspoon brown sugar
- 1 small egg, beaten
- 2 ounces unsalted butter
- 2 teaspoons cornstarch
- 1 sheet puff pastry, thawed or fresh
- 2 cups frozen blueberries

Directions

- Combine blueberries, sugar with the lemon juice and simmer for 10 minutes in a small saucepan.
- Follow by stirring in the butter.
- Make sure to dilute cornstarch in 1 tablespoon of water in a cup.

- Add bit of the blueberry sauce, stir well to mix.
- Pour the cornstarch into the saucepan, make sure to stir until the sauce is thick.
- Pour it into a bowl when ready, let cool for 30 minutes.
- Preheat an oven to 400°F.
- Unfold the puff pastry and roll it out.
- Cut into squares.
- Scoop 2 heaped teaspoons blueberry filling in the middle of pastry squares.
- Run your finger alongside the sides of each square after dipping your finger in water.
- Lift one tip of the pastry and fold it over the filling towards the opposite tip forming a triangle.
- To seal, press down the edges.
- Double-seal with a fork.
- Place turnovers onto a baking tray.
- Pierce each turnover to allow steam to escape.
- Brush with egg wash and sprinkle with brown sugar.
- Bake in the oven for 15 minutes.

- When ready, serve and enjoy.

Strawberry coconut tart

This recipe uses simple and easy to find ingredients. It is quite easy to make from scratch in 35 minutes.

Ingredients

- 2/3 cups of unsweetened desiccated coconut
- 1 stick unsalted butter , melted
- 4 tablespoons of strawberry jam
- 3 tablespoons of powdered sugar
- 1 cup of all-purpose flour
- ½ cup of powdered sugar
- 1 egg white, from a large egg

Directions

- In a mixing bowl, combine flour with powdered sugar.
- Add melted butter.
- Make sure to mix thoroughly with a large spoon.
- Mix your hands when it begins to form dough.
- Wrap it and let chill for 30 minutes.
- Remove it from the fridge and fill the bottom and sides of a pie pan with it. Do not roll.

- Take a piece of the pastry and press it down. This should be piece by piece until you use up all of it.
- Spread jam over the crust. Keep aside.
- Whip the egg white until soft peaks appear.
- Add sifted sugar and beat until smooth.
- Stir in the coconut.
- Pour this mixture over the jam and spread evenly round.
- Bake in a preheated oven at 350°F for 25-30 minutes.
- Remove out when ready and let it cool totally.
- Serve and enjoy.

Hot pink coconut slaw

Ingredients

- ½ cup of chopped cilantro
- 1 cup of large unsweetened coconut flakes
- 2 tablespoons of olive oil
- 1 small jalapeño, seeds and membranes removed, chopped
- 1 cup of thinly sliced radishes
- 1 tablespoon of honey or maple syrup
- ½ teaspoon of salt
- ¼ cup of lime juice
- ¼ cup of apple cider vinegar
- 1 medium red onion, thinly sliced
- 4 cups of thinly sliced purple cabbage

Directions

- In a large serving bowl, combine the lime juice, vinegar, olive oil, honey and salt.
- Add the remaining ingredients and toss to combine.
- Set aside for 20 minutes, tossing occasionally.
- Taste and adjust accordingly.

- Keep for 4 hours.
- Serve and enjoy.

Almond coconut granola bars

Ingredients

- 1 cup of chopped almonds
- ½ cup of honey or maple syrup
- ½ teaspoon of salt
- 1 ¾ of cups quick-cooking oats
- 1 cup of creamy almond butter
- 1 ½ teaspoons of vanilla extract
- 1 cup large of unsweetened coconut flakes
- ½ teaspoon of ground cinnamon

Directions

- Start by lining a square baker with two strips of crisscrossed parchment paper, cut to fit neatly against the base and up the sides.
- In a medium skillet over medium heat, toast the almonds, stirring frequently, until they are fragrant and starting to turn lightly golden on the edges in 5 minutes.
- Transfer them to a medium mixing bowl.

- To the mixing bowl, add the oats together with the coconut flakes, cinnamon and salt. Stir to blended.
- In a 2-cup liquid measuring cup, add 1 cup almond butter.
- Top with ½ cup honey, then add the vanilla extract.
- Whisk until well blended.
- Mix the liquid ingredients with the dry ingredients.
- Mix them together using a sizeable spoon until the two are evenly combined and no dry oats remain.
- Shift the mixture to the prepared square baker.
- Use your spoon to organize the mixture fairly evenly in the baker, then use the bottom of a flat, round surface to pack the mixture down as firmly and evenly as possible.
- Then, cover the baker and refrigerate for more than 1 hour and let the oats absorb moisture so the granola bars can set.

- Lift the bars out of the baker by grabbing both pieces of parchment paper on opposite corners.
- Using a sharp knife, slice the mixture into 4 even rows and 4 even columns.
- Serve and enjoy.
- These bars can last well for a couple of days at room temperature.

Tex-Mex breakfast bowls

Ingredients

For Pico de Gallo

- 1 tablespoon of lime juice
- 1 pint of cherry or grape tomatoes, quartered
- ¼ teaspoon of fine-grain sea salt
- ¼ cup of chopped fresh cilantro
- ¼ cup of finely chopped white onion

For the Refried black beans

- ½ teaspoon of garlic powder.
- ½ teaspoon of fine-grain sea salt
- 1 tablespoon olive oil
- 1 teaspoon of lime juice
- ½ cup finely chopped white onion
- 2 teaspoons of ground cumin
- Freshly ground black pepper
- 2 cans of black beans, rinsed and drained
- ½ cup of water

For the scrambled eggs

- 10 eggs
- 3 tablespoons of cream

- ¼ teaspoon of fine-grain sea salt
- Freshly ground black pepper
- Pinch of pepper flakes
- 2 teaspoons of olive oil
- ½ cup of grated Monterey Jack cheese or cheddar cheese

For everything else

- Roasted breakfast potatoes
- 1 ripe avocado, thinly sliced
- Your favorite salsa

Directions

- In a small mixing bowl, combine grated tomatoes, white onion, cilantro, lime juice and sea salt stir to combine, keep to marinate.
- In a medium saucepan over medium heat, warm the olive oil until shimmering but with no smoke.
- Add the chopped onion and a sprinkle of salt.
- Let cook as you keep, stirring occasionally, until the onion turning translucent in 8 minutes.
- Add the cumin together with the garlic.

- Let cook until fragrant in 30 seconds, stirring occasionally.
- Pour in the drained beans and water. Stir, cover and cook for 5 minutes.
- Lower the heat and mash up at least half of the beans.
- Let continue to cook uncovered, stirring often, for 3 more minutes.
- Remove the saucepan from the heat and stir in the salt, pepper and lime juice.
- Taste and adjust accordingly.
- Cover until you're ready to serve.
- In another separate medium mixing bowl, scramble the eggs with the cream, salt, a few twists of freshly ground black pepper and a pinch of red pepper flakes.
- In a non-stick, warm 2 teaspoons olive oil over medium heat until shimmering without smoke.
- Swirl the pan to evenly coated with oil.
- Then, whisk your egg mixture one last time and pour into the skillet.

- Scramble the eggs by pushing the mixture around until 90 percent set.
- Remove the pan from the heat source, stir in the cheese.
- Divide the beans and scrambled eggs evenly into 4 bowls.
- Stir the Pico de Gallo again, and use a slotted spoon to divide the Pico de Gallo into the bowls.
- Leave the watery tomato juice in the bowl.
- Top each bowl with a few slices of thinly sliced avocado.
- Serve and enjoy with a salsa of your choice.

Clumpy granola with stewed rhubarb

Ingredients

- 2 tablespoons of maple syrup
- ½ cup of almonds, chopped
- ½ cup of puffed brown rice
- ½ cup of chickpea flour
- 1 vanilla bean pod, scraped
- ¼ cup of pepitas
- 2 rhubarb stalks, trimmed and cut pieces
- ¼ cup of sunflower seeds
- 1 teaspoon of ground cinnamon
- 2 cups of old-fashioned oats
- 2 teaspoons of lemon juice
- 1 teaspoon of ground ginger
- ½ teaspoon of ground nutmeg
- ½ teaspoon of sea salt
- Scant ½ cup of maple syrup
- Scant ½ cup of melted coconut oil

Directions

- Start by preheating your oven to 300°F, then line a large baking sheet with parchment paper.

- Next, in a large mixing bowl, combine the oats together with the almonds, puffed rice, sunflower seeds, chickpea flour, pumpkin seeds, nutmeg, cinnamon, ginger, and salt. Mix to blend.

- In another smaller bowl, whisk together the maple syrup and coconut oil until combined.

- Pour the wet mixture into the dry, and mix well.

- Move the granola to the prepared baking sheet and use the back of a big spoon to spread it out into an even layer.

- Let bake for about 40 minutes, rotating the pan halfway through, until golden and fragrant.

- Allow the pan to cool completely to keep the clumps intact.

- Gently break up the granola into clumps and store in an airtight container at room temperature for up to 2 weeks or in a freezer.
- Then, heat a medium saucepan over medium-low heat.
- Add the rhubarb together with the maple syrup, lemon juice, and vanilla bean, and stir to mix.
- Cover let cook for 10 minutes, stirring occasionally, until the mixture is bubbling and the rhubarb is tender. Keep aside for later.
- Divide the yogurt between 4 bowls
- Then, add ½ cup granola to each bowl and then divide the stewed rhubarb into the bowls.
- Serve and enjoy.

Blueberry baked oatmeal

Ingredients

- 2 teaspoons of raw sugar
- 2 teaspoons of ground cinnamon
- 12 ounces of fresh or frozen blueberries
- 1 teaspoon baking powder
- Vanilla yogurt
- ¾ teaspoon of fine-grain sea salt
- ¼ teaspoon of ground nutmeg
- ⅔ cup of roughly chopped pecans
- 1 ¾ cups of milk of choice
- ⅓ cup of maple syrup or honey
- 2 large eggs or flax eggs
- 2 cups of old-fashioned oats
- 3 tablespoons of melted unsalted butter
- 2 teaspoons of vanilla extract

Directions

- Expressly, preheat your oven ready to 375°F.
- Then, oil a square baking dish .

- Pour the nuts onto a rimmed baking sheet when the oven has finished preheating, let toast for 5 minutes, until fragrant.
- In a medium mixing bowl, combine the oats together with the, toasted nuts, cinnamon, baking powder, salt and nutmeg. Mix to combine.
- In another separate smaller mixing bowl, combine the milk, maple syrup, egg, half of the butter, and vanilla. Mix until blended.
- Reserve about ½ cup of the berries for topping the baked oatmeal, then arrange the remaining berries evenly over the bottom of the baking dish
- Cover the fruit with the dry oat mixture, then drizzle the wet ingredients over the oats.
- Wiggle the baking dish to make sure the milk moves down through the oats, then gently pat down any dry oats resting on top.
- Scatter the remaining berries across the top.
- Sprinkle some raw sugar on top for extra sweetness and crunch.

- Let bake for 45 minutes, until the top is nice and golden.
- Remove your baked oatmeal from the oven.
- Allow it to cool for briefly for few minutes.
- Then, drizzle with the remaining melted butter on the top.
- Serve and enjoy.
- Any left overs can be kept in the fridge for up to 5 days.

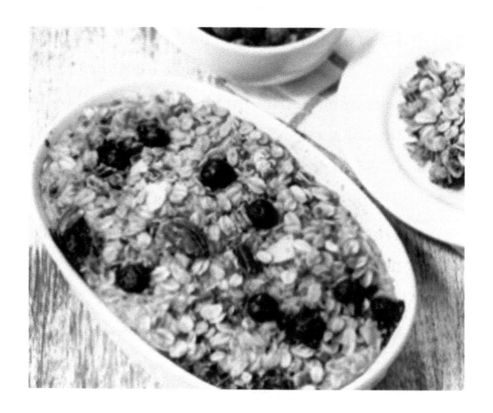

Healthy carrot muffins

Ingredients

- ½ cup of maple syrup or honey
- 1 teaspoon of ground cinnamon
- ½ teaspoon of salt
- 1 tablespoon of turbinado sugar
- ⅓ cup of melted coconut oil
- ½ teaspoon of ground ginger
- 1 teaspoon of vanilla extract
- ¼ teaspoon of ground nutmeg
- 1 ¾ cups of white whole wheat flour
- 1 cup of plain Greek yogurt
- 2 eggs, preferably at room temperature
- 1 ½ teaspoons of baking powder
- ½ teaspoon of baking soda
- 2 cups of peeled and grated carrots
- ½ cup of roughly chopped walnuts
- ½ cup of raisins tossed in 1 teaspoon flour

Directions

- Preheat oven to 425°F.

- Grease all the 12 cups on the muffin tin with butter.
- In a large mixing bowl, combine the flour together with the baking powder, cinnamon, baking soda, salt, ginger and nutmeg. Blend with a whisk.
- In a separate, small bowl, toss the raisins with 1 teaspoon flour to avoid sticking together.
- Add the grated carrots together with the chopped walnuts and floured raisins to the other ingredients and stir to combine.
- In another separated medium sized mixing bowl, combine the oil and maple syrup, let whisk together.
- Add the eggs and beat well, then add the yogurt together with vanilla, mix well.
- Mix the wet ingredients together with the dry ones then mix with a big spoon, to combine.
- Divide the batter evenly between the 12 muffin cups.
- Sprinkle the tops of the muffins with turbinado sugar.

- Let bake for 16 minutes, until the muffins are golden on top and a toothpick inserted into a muffin comes out clean.
- Place the muffin tin on a cooling rack to cool.
- Serve and enjoy.
- The muffins when frozen, can last for up to 3 months.

Cranberry orange granola bars

Ingredients

- ¾ teaspoon of salt
- 1 cup of pecan pieces
- 1 ½ teaspoons of vanilla extract
- ⅔ cup of dried cranberries
- ½ cup of honey
- 1 ¾ cups of quick-cooking oats
- 1 teaspoon of orange zest, preferably organic
- 1 cup of creamy unsalted almond butter or peanut butter, packed
- ½ teaspoon of ground cinnamon
- ⅓ cup of pepitas

Directions

- Firstly, line a square baker with two strips of crisscrossed parchment paper, cut to fit neatly against the base and up the sides.
- In a medium skillet over medium heat, toast the pecans and pepitas, stirring often, until they are fragrant in 5 minutes.

- Move the toasted pecans and pepitas to a food processor.
- Then, add the cranberries and then run the machine for about 10 seconds, until the nuts and cranberries are all broken up.
- In a mixing bowl, combine the contents of the food processor together with the oats, orange zest, cinnamon and salt. Mix to combine.
- In another separate smaller mixing bowl, mix together the almond butter, honey and vanilla extract until well blended.
- Mix the liquid ingredients together with the dry ingredients.
- Use a big spoon to mix them together until the two are evenly combined and no dry oats remain.
- Shift the mixture to the prepared square baker.
- By the Use of a spoon, arrange the mixture fairly evenly in the baker.
- Then, use the bottom of a flat, round surface covered in a small piece of parchment paper,

to pack the mixture down as firmly and evenly as possible.

- Cover the baker and refrigerate for 2 hours or overnight for the best outcome.
- To slice, lift the bars out of the baker by grabbing both pieces of parchment paper on opposite corners.
- With a sharp knife, slice the bars into strips, then slice them in half through the middle.
- Serve and enjoy.
- Any left overs can be kept in the fridge for days.

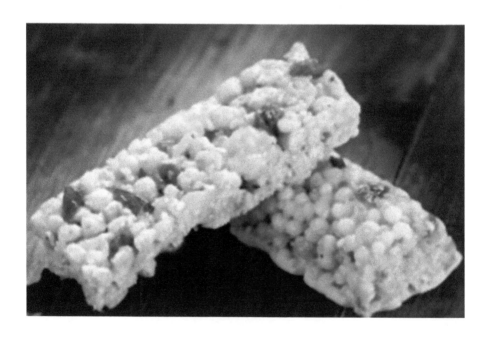

Butternut squash frittata with fried sage

Ingredients

- Freshly ground black pepper
- 16 fresh sage leaves
- 2 cloves garlic
- ¾ cup of freshly grated Parmesan
- 3 tablespoons of extra-virgin olive oil
- 8 eggs
- ¾ pound of butternut squash
- ½ cup of milk
- ¾ cup of chopped yellow onion
- ¾ teaspoon of sea salt, divided

Directions

- Preheat the oven ready to 425°F.
- In a large bowl, whisk together the eggs together with the milk, garlic, teaspoon salt, and several twists of freshly ground black pepper and half of the cheese.
- In a well-seasoned cast iron skillet, warm 1 tablespoon olive oil over medium heat.
- Add the chopped onion, stir to coat.

- Let cook for a few minutes, until the onions are starting to turn translucent.
- Add the squash and ½ teaspoon salt and stir to mix.
- Cover the pan and reduce heat, let cook for 8 minutes as you stir occasionally.
- Uncover the pan, raise the heat back to medium continue to cook until the excess moisture has evaporated in about 6 or 10 minutes.
- Lower the heat.
- Arrange the butternut in an even layer in the bottom of the skillet.
- Then, whisk the egg mixture one last time and pour it into the pan.
- Sprinkle the frittata with the remaining cheese.
- Put the pan in the oven and bake until you can shake the pan and you can the middle is just barely set in 17 minutes.
- Then, heat oil in a large skillet over medium heat.

- Once the oil is shimmering, add the sage and toss to coat.
- Let the sage get crispy then transferring it to a plate covered with a paper towel.
- Sprinkle the fried sage lightly with sea salt and set it aside.
- Sprinkle fried sage on top and let the frittata rest a few minutes, then slice into 8 smaller wedges.
- Serve and enjoy.

Mango panna cotta

Though a perfect Mediterranean Sea diet, mango panna cotta an Italian desert wonderful picnics, parties and dinners. It can be prepared ahead of time.

Ingredients

- A knob of butter
- ½ cup of whole milk
- ½ teaspoon of vanilla essence
- 1 cup of heavy cream the whole package
- 1 packet gelatin
- ½ lemon, juice only
- 2 cups of frozen mango chunks, thawed
- ⅓ cup of granulated sugar
- 2 tablespoons of granulated sugar

Directions

- Pour heavy cream together with the milk and sugar into a small sauce pan.
- Stir to dissolve the sugar on over low heat, the cream should be hot.
- Turn off the heat and stir vanilla essence. Make sure not to boil at this stage.

- The bloom should be gelatin as per the package Directions.
- Add the bloomed gelatin to the cooled cream mixture. Do not forget to mix to dissolve.
- Pour the mixture into small glasses, place to refrigerate to set the panna cotta for 2 hours.
- Process the thawed mango pieces together with the lemon juice and sugar in a blender until smooth.
- Taste and adjust accordingly.
- Simmer in a small saucepan over low heat.
- Stir in butter to get a much creamier texture.
- Allow the mixture to cool.
- Pour over the panna cotta.
- Serve and enjoy.

Candied oranges dipped in chocolate

This recipe is for a sweet tasty treat for a perfect holiday to enjoy Mediterranean Sea diet. The chocolates can be substituted with cupcakes if you like.

Ingredients

- 3.5 ounces of Dark Chocolate
- 1 Large Orange, organic
- Coarse Salt
- 1 cup of Granulated Sugar
- 1 cup of Water

Directions

- Cut the oranges into thin slices.
- Heat water and sugar in a large pot until the sugar has dissolved.
- Add the orange slices in a manner that they are spread around without covering each other totally.
- Let simmer for 40 minutes on a low heat. Turn occasionally.
- Transfer slices onto a wire rack when ready, let them cool completely.

- It is fine to cool on a fridge to speed up the cooling process.
- Melt the chocolate over a pot of simmering water.
- Dip half of each slice in chocolate.
- Place the dipped one's onto a tray lined with a sheet of aluminum foil.
- Sprinkle with salt.
- Shift all of them into the fridge.
- Serve an enjoy.

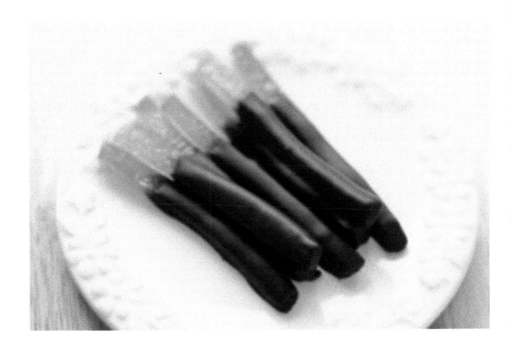

Walnut crescent cookies

If you want taste and know divine taste covered in a powdered sugar, look no further, walnut crescent cookies can give you that same exact taste.

Ingredients

- 2 tablespoons of vanilla sugar
- 11/4 cup of all-purpose flour
- ½ cup of powdered sugar
- 1 stick unsalted butter
- ⅔ cup of ground walnuts
- 4 tablespoons of powdered sugar
- 1 teaspoon of vanilla essence

Directions

- In a large mixing bowl, begin by combining sifted powdered sugar, sifted flour, and ground walnuts.
- Next, add vanilla essence and mix thoroughly.
- Then, grate chilled butter.
- Add to the bowl.

- Combine all the ingredients using your bare hands until dough is formed in 3 minutes or so.
- Place into a Ziploc bag allow it to chill for 30 minutes in the fridge.
- As it refrigerates, get a small bowl and place extra powdered sugar with vanilla sugar in it and keep aside.
- Take a piece of the dough and roll into a ball then into a sausage.
- Shape the sausage into a crescent.
- Place onto a baking tray with baking parchment.
- For the remaining dough, repeat this step.
- Bake in a ready heated oven at 400°F for 8 minutes or so.
- Allow it to cool down completely on the tray when already fried.
- Transfer to a plat and dip with powdered sugar to coat.
- Serve and enjoy.

Caramel apple dip

The caramel apple dip is a perfect and excellent choice for family gatherings with only 3 ingredients, it is a quickie in only 2 minutes with absolutely no cooking and frying needed.

Ingredients

- Caramels
- ½ cup of Dulce de leche
- 2 – 3 apples, cut into small pieces
- ½ cup of cream cheese

Directions

- In a bowl, mix the cream cheese together with the Dulce de leech until smooth.
- Cut the apples into quarters after rinsing.
- Remove the hard parts.
- Further cut every quarter into 6 slices
- Serve and enjoy.

Easy lemon cupcakes

Lemon is a nutritious fruit fantastic for a Mediterranean Sea diet. The lemon gives this recipe a flavorful taste super moist topped with vanilla mascarpone cream cheese frosting.

Ingredients

- ½ cup of granulated sugar
- 3/4 cup of all-purpose flour
- 2 eggs, at room temperature
- 2 teaspoon of baking powder
- 1/4 teaspoon of vanilla essence
- 3 small lemons, juice only
- A pinch of salt
- ½ cup of powdered sugar
- 1 tablespoon of lemon juice
- 1 stick unsalted butter , softened
- 9 ounces of mascarpone cheese
- ½ cup of cream cheese

Directions

- Firstly, begin by preheating your oven to 360°F.

- Juice all the lemons without the seeds, keep for later.
- In a mixing dish, beat the butter together with sugar until creamy in 3 minutes.
- Add the eggs and mix well.
- Combine the flour together with the baking powder and salt.
- Add this to the cupcake batter and mix until smooth.
- Pour in the lemon juice and mix thoroughly for the last time.
- Place the paper cases in a muffin tray.
- Using a pipe, pipe the batter into paper cases.
- Let bake for 15 minutes.
- If you the inserted skewer comes out clean, it is an indication that the cupcakes are ready.
- Remove from the oven.
- Pour in the balance of the lemon juice over each cupcake (2 spoons per cake).
- Allow it to cool down completely.
- Shift all the ingredients into a mixing bowl.

- Combine them using an electric mixer until smooth.
- Serve and enjoy.

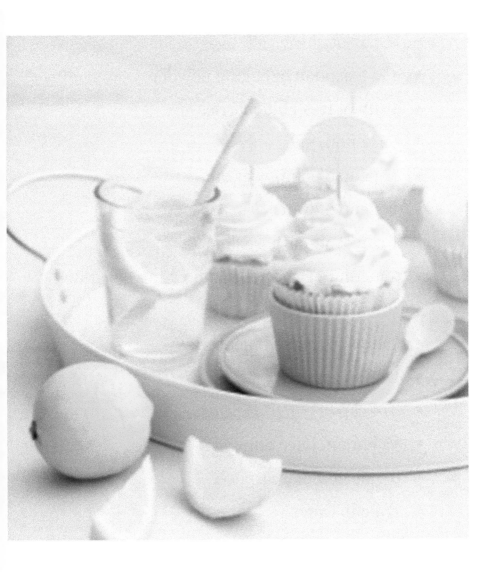

Lemon blueberry poke cake from scratch

This is a typical moist sponge soft recipe featuring blueberry sauce and creamy ricotta with a hint of lemon to give it the attractive flavor for a Mediterranean Sea diet.

Ingredients

- ½ cup of powdered sugar
- 1½ teaspoon of baking powder
- 1 cup of fresh blueberries
- ½ lemon, juice only
- 1/4 cup of sunflower oil
- 1/4 cup of water
- 1 cup of all-purpose flour
- 3 medium eggs, yolks and whites separated
- ½ cup of granulated sugar
- 2 cups of frozen blueberries
- Lemon zest
- 3/4 cup of granulated sugar
- ½ lemon, juice only
- 8 ounce of mascarpone
- 1/4 cup water
- 8 ounce of ricotta

Directions

- Start by beating the egg whites until soft peaks forms, keep for later.
- In another separate mixing dish, whisk the egg yolks together with sugar until creamy.
- Sift in flour mixed with baking powder. Mix properly.
- Add oil together with water, continue to mix with an electric mixer until smooth.
- Fold in the egg whites and pour the batter in a rectangular baking dish.
- Begin baking for 15 minutes at 375°F.
- Allow it to cool down.
- Pierce in holes when completely cooled.
- As the cake is in the oven, heat up the blueberries together with the water, sugar, and lemon juice in a sauce pan.
- Over low heat simmer for 7 minutes.
- Turn off heat, keep aside.
- In another separate bowl, combine ricotta together with the freshly squeezed lemon juice, mascarpone, and sugar.

- Place in the electric mixer mix until well combined.
- Pour the blueberries and their juice over the cake sponge.
- Then, spread the ricotta layer over.
- Refrigerate to chill.
- Serve and enjoy with blueberries and or grated lemon zest if you like.

Chocolate mango cheesecake parfait

This is an excellent choice for passing through the summer season. It combines Oreo cookies with fresh mangoes, mango cheesecake and chocolate for a tastier breakfast for a Mediterranean diet.

Ingredients

- 3 tablespoons of lemon juice
- 1 fresh mango
- 12 ounces of cream cheese
- 1 packet of Oreo cookies
- ½ cup of whipping cream
- 2 tablespoons of unsweetened cocoa powder
- ½ cup of powdered sugar

Instruction

- Begin by cutting the mango, scoop the flesh from one half out.
- Puree in a food processor, keep aside.
- The remaining half should be cut into slices.
- Whip the cream until soft peaks form in a small mixing dish.

- Add the cream cheese together with the powdered sugar and mix to combined.
- Divide this mixture equally between 2 dishes.
- Add pureed mango and lemon juice in one.
- Fill the next one with cocoa powder.
- Mix both until well combined.
- You can start with a whole Oreo cookie.
- Then a mango cheesecake layer, fresh mango slices.
- Then, lastly, place the chocolate cheesecake layer.
- Repeat this until everything is finished.
- Garnish with some Oreo crumb.
- Refrigerate for 1 hour to chill.
- Serve and enjoy.

Mango tiramisu

This a Mediterranean delicious fruity version of the Italian classic desert. It features mango sauce, mascarpone mixture and layers of ladyfingers finished with cocoa or mango slices in 30 minutes.

Ingredients

- 12 ounce of mascarpone cheese
- 9 ounce of sour cream
- 1 cup of hot water
- 1/4 cup of water
- 2 teaspoons of instant coffee
- 4 tablespoons of vanilla sugar
- 2 cups of fresh mango pieces
- 5 tablespoons of granulated sugar
- ½ medium lemon, juice only
- 7 ounce of ladyfingers

Directions

- Mix your coffee with hot water in a jug. Allow it to cool down in totality.
- As the coffee cooling, put diced mango in a sauce pan

- Add sugar and water.
- Over low heat, simmer the mixture for 4 minutes.
- Turn off the heat.
- Shift the content into a bowl, add juice from half a lemon
- Using a fork, mash the mango. Stir and let it cool down.
- Combine the mascarpone together with the sour cream and vanilla sugar in a dish.
- Mix this until smooth, preferably using an electric mixer.
- Get a loaf tin and line it with aluminum foil.
- Pour the coffee into a shallow plate.
- Immediately dip each ladyfinger in it.
- Cover the whole bottom of the tin with ladyfingers.
- Spread over about a third of the mascarpone mixture.
- Top with chilled mango sauce.
- Repeat until everything is done.

- Refrigerate the tiramisu in a fridge for at 3 hours.
- Dust the top with cocoa powder.

Serve and enjoy with mango slices garnished on top.

Raspberry mint ice pops

Mint is one element in this recipe that gives it a refreshing taste and keeping you hooked onto it. The raspberry flavor can be felt through the entire raspberry.

Ingredients

- 1½ cup of Fresh Raspberries
- 1 Wedge of Lemon
- ⅓ cup of Honey
- 10 Mint Leaves
- 1 cup of Water

Directions

- In a small sauce pan, combine the honey, water, together with 5 mint leaves.
- Heat this up without boiling until the honey is melted. Keep for later.
- Then, puree the raspberries including the remaining mint leaves in a food processor.
- Sieve the mixture to remove any seeds in it.
- Make sure to remove any mint leaves from honey water at this stage.
- Add in the pureed raspberries.

- Squeeze in the lemon mix thoroughly.
- Then pour it into popsicle molds.
- Freeze for at least 8 hours, otherwise 12 hours is best.
- Serve and enjoy.

Honey lemony ricotta breakfast toast with figs and pistachios

Ingredients

- ¼ cup of low fat ricotta
- 2 tablespoons of pistachio pieces
- 1 teaspoon of lemon zest
- ½ fresh of lemon, juiced
- ½ tablespoon of honey
- 2 slices whole grain
- 4 figs, sliced

Directions

- Toast bread in toaster.
- Whip together ricotta, lemon juice and honey until smooth and creamy.
- Spread ricotta moisture evenly over each piece of toast.
- Top with sliced figs.
- Sprinkle each piece with pistachio pieces and lemon zest.
- Serve and enjoy.

Mango yogurt popsicles

This is per harps the most refreshing Mediterranean Sea diet healthiest mango drink with simple and easy to make ingredients. It is also perfect for the summer.

Ingredients

- 1 stick of <u>unsalted butter</u>
- 5 ounces of milk chocolate
- 1 cup of <u>Greek yogurt</u>
- 1 wedge lemon
- 1/4 cup of <u>granulated sugar</u>
- 2½ cups of frozen mango pieces, slightly thawed

Directions

- Combine the yogurt together with lemon juice, sugar, and mango pieces in a food processor.
- Process until smooth.
- Pour the mixture in a popsicle mold with inserted sticks.
- Place in the freezer overnight.
- Remove the popsicles, allow then to heat to room temperature for a few minutes.

- Take out of the molds.
- Place a sheet of parchment paper in the freezer and place the popsicles onto it.
- Cut the chocolate into tiny pieces, place all of them a dish.
- Add diced butter and melt over a double boiler.
- Pour this melted chocolate into mug that is preferably heat proof for dipping each popsicle.
- As you take out, allow the excess chocolate to gently drip back.
- Make sure to repeat this very step with all the reaming popsicles.
- Place the ready ones back in the freezer.
- Remove, let settle to a bit.
- Serve and enjoy.

Lightning Source UK Ltd.
Milton Keynes UK
UKHW020746030621
384855UK00001B/162